Investment Guide for Doctors

Steve Petty, M.D.

Copyright © 2022 Steve Petty

All rights reserved.

ISBN:

ISBN-13:

Contents

Dedication	v
Preface	vii
Disclaimer	ix
1. Retirement Investing 101	1
2. Free Financial Advice: Mind Your Own Business	5
3. Debt-to-Income Ratio	11
4. Beating the Market	15
5. Predicting Stock Market Direction	21
6. Index Investing	23
7. The Great Recession	27
8. Is Your Money Safe?	31
9. The 1% Home Loan	35
10. Playing Defense	39
11. Fundamentals of Asset Allocation	43
12. Mad Money: Picking Individual Stocks	45
13. Getting Whipsawed	49
14. Margin Management: Using Leverage	53
15. A Financial, Personal, and Legacy Retirement Plan	59
16. Banks and Savings	65
17. Market Booms and Busts	69
18. Diversification	73
19. Getting Good Investment Advice	77
20. Real Estate Riches: Why Not Become a Slum Lord?	81
21. Savings: The Heart of Investing	85
22. Spending Power: Personal Finance 101	89
23. Can Decluttering Make You Wealthy?	93
About the Author	99
Other Books by the Author	101

Dedication

To the men and women at Kaiser Permanente, dedicating their lives daily to their patients, community, and families. And especially to Suzanne Yokoyama and Haritha Rachamallu, who originally asked me to write most of these articles to our physicians in our quarterly newsletter, *Connects the Docs*.

Preface

Investment Guide for Doctors consists of articles written between 2005 and 2015 for Kaiser Permanente physicians (and anyone else with a regular paycheck) in a newsletter called *Connect the Docs*.

Much of these lessons are common sense—living below your means, making automatic withdrawals from your paycheck to invest in your 401k, maintaining an emergency fund of six months of living expenses, and being your own financial advisor. After I wrote about ten of the articles, one of the editors asked me to put the articles together in a book so everything would be available in one place. That was my goal for this book: to compile them all.

I must admit that my investing resume is quite sketchy. I've bought and sold stocks and mutual funds, exchange-traded funds and stock options, and bought and sold rental real estate. One time about ten years ago, after selling and buying 200 stocks and option trades, I called my broker to ask a question.

Preface

She told me that I qualified for a $2 discount on all my future trades because I was a *high-volume trader*. A "silver trader" is what she called me. Then I started getting notices from my brokerage firm, accusing me of day trading.

I've also used leverage, borrowing money from my home equity line of credit to invest in the stock market, and then borrowing money from the broker on that borrowed money to buy market index exchange traded funds on steroids—volatile and insomnia producing, especially in a down market.

It's been my pleasure to help friends, family, and colleagues (none of them went broke or filed bankruptcy), but I've never been so humbled or learned so much by getting my butt kicked in the stock market and in real estate.

The truth is that I contracted the investing bug. I read more than 200 investment books. I purchased magazines like *Fortune, Money, Kiplinger's,* and *Baron's,* and I have subscriptions to *Bob Brinker's Market Timer, Investor's Business Daily, Vector Vest,* and *Gorilla Trades*. I was at one time smitten with investment shows like *Mad Money* with host Jim Cramer, whose books are quite entertaining as well. I also watched nightly business reports like *Fast Money*. I sat with my black notebook opened, taking notes and writing the ticker symbols, looking for stock picks. I've had many teachers throughout my journey.

My hope is that you'll find this book helpful as you navigate through the investment jungle. If you're a doctor, just never forget that "M.D." doesn't mean "medical doctor" to a financial advisor. It means "more dough" for them.

Happy Investing!

Steve

Disclaimer

The views and opinions of the physician authors expressed in the *Connect the Docs* newsletter are those of the authors alone and do not necessarily state or reflect those of Kaiser Permanente. The financial information is not designed to counsel individual investors but only to inform and educate. Those seeking specific investment advice should consider a qualified investment professional.

1. Retirement Investing 101

"Often when you think you're at the end of something, you're at the beginning of something else."

— Fred Rogers

Money, Health, Activities, Friends, and Family

My cousin who retired eight years ago asked me during a family dinner last month, "What are you going to do when you retire?" Interesting. I'd never thought about it. My former physician in chief, Dr. Blair Beebe, wrote a book. Dr. Roger Lake volunteered in a free clinic. Dr. Greg Denari planned to teach medical students in Aruba. Dr. Steve Henry, a retired urologist, traveled the country while working as a locum tenens. I told my cousin I might play more guitar and sing and maybe buy a bus and go on tour with the band I play in, Petty Therapy.

I thought retirement was all about having the proper financial

Retirement Investing 101

preparation and strategies, but according to Richard Stim and Ralph Warner's book *Retire Happy*, "The most powerful predictor of life satisfaction after retirement is the size of your social network." It wasn't a coincidence that my happily retired cousin was sitting with me and twelve other family members after we had all watched my twelve-year-old nephew's basketball game. The family ate dinner together, laughed and joked, and had a good time. I don't think my cousin read the book *Retire Happy*, but she understood that there's more to retirement than financial planning. Retirement research has helped me understand the importance of making sound financial investments, but it's also essential to invest in your health, friends, and hobbies.

Here are some basics to consider:

Money: There are basically three financial assets you should keep track of and accumulate over your career: your 401k, your IRA, and your cash. The 401k and IRA may have stocks, mutual funds, or bonds in them. A colleague emailed and asked if he should max out his 401k. Yes! Yes! Yes! It's free money. 401k money isn't taxed until we take money out in retirement, and by then most of us will be in a lower tax bracket. Add retirement savings to an IRA even if it isn't tax deductible. Try to live below your means and save some cash each month.

Get out of credit card debt and pay the balance every month. Have a plan to pay off your house by the time you retire. Meet with at least two financial planners… at least one with Fidelity and your own private financial planner.

Health: I know many of you doctors recommend regular exercise, but do you do it yourself? The benefits of exercise are enormous. Remember that thirty minutes of walking or other aerobic exercise daily is also a great way to manage stress.

Obese and overweight people make up two-thirds of the US population. Are you in the overweight bracket? Keep your weight down. You know all the benefits—less arthritis, heart disease, hypertension, etc.

How is your diet? Make a habit of eating healthy food now so it's easier to keep the momentum going in your later years. Get your cholesterol and blood pressure checked. Invest the time and effort in your health now so you can enjoy a healthy retirement.

Friends and Family: Most of us plan financially for retirement, but do we really plan or develop a network of friends and keep in contact with them? It's the most important aspect of a satisfying retirement according to some studies. Some plan to spend more time with grandkids. Don't forget pets. According to one of my doctor colleagues, people with a dog tend to live longer, and pets have been known to lower blood pressure. Invest some time at social gatherings with people you like and may hang out with in the future. Spend time with people who enjoy a similar hobby. That might be golfing, hiking, biking, or BBQ-ing.

Hobbies: Remember time, not money, is really life's most important asset. According to Social Security data, a woman who survives to sixty-five is likely to live another twenty years; a man who survives to sixty-five will live another fifteen years. The average retirement age is sixty-three for a man and sixty-two for a woman. According to the CDC, the average life expectancy for Americans in the year 2022 is seventy-seven years old.

So what do you plan to do with your time? Engage in enjoyable activities? Do you even have hobbies that you enjoy? Travel, writing, music, volunteering? Attending ballets, concerts, symphonies? Or maybe you want to work part time. You won't be able to work with the medical group after you retire, but you can work somewhere else.

I always thought retirement meant the end of our regular life, but it's really only the beginning of a new phase. Investing in finances for retirement is important. Consider investing some time and energy in your health, social network, and activities—in addition to your finances. I never really thought about what I would do after the magic day when I stopped working, until my very happily retired cousin asked me at our family's get together, "What are you going to do when you retire?" How about you?

Four important areas to invest in now for a quality retirement:
– Money
– Health
– Friends and family
– Hobbies

2. Free Financial Advice: Mind Your Own Business

"One of the hardest things about wealth building is to be true to yourself and be willing to not go along with the crowd."

— Robert Kiyosaki, author of *Rich Dad Poor Dad*

In his book *Rich Dad Poor Dad*, Robert Kiyosaki wrote that it's very important to mind your own business. I think it's important to mind our own business because we're all taxed like a business. One of the most important decisions anyone makes is to manage their own personal finances. There are sharks eating innocent investors retirement plans for breakfast, lunch, and dinner. If you think that just because you have "M.D." after your name you're protected, you're wrong. In fact, that "M.D." behind your name is like blood to a shark—it makes the financial advisors and planners hungry for your business. They have kids, too, who need to go to college.

Celebrities are notoriously poor personal financial managers.

Free Financial Advice: Mind Your Own Business

Mike Tyson, a former professional boxer, filed bankruptcy after earning $300 million during his career. Alan Iverson, a former professional basketball player, earned $150 million and had to file bankruptcy. M.C. Hammer, the rap singer from Fremont, California, filed for bankruptcy after earning $10 million in one year. When an interviewer asked why he had to file, he replied, "I made $10 million and paid out $15 million. You do the math."

These high earners all ignored their personal finances. In other words, they didn't mind their own business. They could have prevented those bankruptcies by managing their money properly.

I suggest that you become your own financial advisor. You should also use financial services and get advice, but you must have the last word in managing your money.

Before consulting a financial advisor, consider the following steps, which are low-risk ways to mind your own business:

1. **Define your financial goals** – Retirement, college for kids… Make a plan for those goals. Failure to plan is one common reason people don't reach their goals.
2. **Know what your income and expenses are monthly** – You must keep track. Don't leave this to someone else, or someone else may take some of it. Make sure you live within your means. Don't overextend your expenses with a house you can't afford. Don't live a rich-and-famous lifestyle, spending more than you make. Living paycheck to paycheck is a formula for only survival, not for success.
3. **Protect your cash flow** – Keep an emergency cash fund—six to twenty-four months—of living expenses in case of emergencies. Consider disability insurance

in case you become unable to work. Also, consider life insurance if you have kids or dependents. Some advisors suggest protecting your cash flow by investing in annuities so you can receive dividend income from dividend stocks or mutual funds. Others suggest using a bond ladder. The problem is that you have to pay for all of those, and they all carry more risk. But then even saving cash is risky if inflation hits.
4. **Tax strategies** – Maximize your investment in your 401k. It's a good way to save for retirement, and you aren't taxed on the money until you take it out. Most people are in a lower tax bracket when they retire, so they pay less taxes when they make both deposits and withdraws. And your home mortgage interest is still tax deductible.
5. **Know your assets and liabilities** – You should create an annual net-worth statement so you have a robust picture of your financial health.

Once you have taken these five steps, consider seeing a financial planner and keep these things in mind:

Be sure to ask how they get paid – They may get a percentage of your portfolio (usually 1% to 2% a year, and that's on top of mutual fund fees). Or they may

Free Financial Advice: Mind Your Own Business

offer a set-fee service for the one to two hours you spend with them. They might also sell you things like insurance and annuities for a commission.

Understand why they are motivated to be your financial planner – When your financial planner smiles, you might see large shark teeth. They usually have their own interests in mind. Ask about their investment strategy and about asset allocation. And do some homework before you meet (that includes taking the five steps listed above). Just be aware that they might not be able to help, depending on the type of "advisor" they are.

One of my friends received a $400,000 injury settlement when he wasn't able to work. He saw a financial advisor, who suggested that he purchase $200,000 in dividend-paying stocks and invest the remaining $200,000 in laddered CDs. Each of these would give him a dividend and some cash flow every three months. But the advisor didn't figure out how much he needed monthly to live on! There's no guarantee that those dividends will support him. Because my friend had signed a contract to keep the money with that "financial advisor," he may be penalized if he needs to take funds out because he's low on cash. He doesn't even have an emergency fund. My friend was financial shark bait, and a shark disguised as a financial advisor gobbled him up.

Understand that there's no guarantee on any investments, and you can always lose money. I got into doing my own financial investments because the first year I invested in a mutual fund recommended by a financial advisor, it lost 58%. Plus, I had to pay expenses to the mutual fund company that lost my money. Some deal, eh? I figured I could do at least as well as they had done if I just paid attention. So can you!

If you want to be your own financial manager, at least take the no-brainer basic steps listed above. No one will manage your money as well as you can. When financial sharks see "M.D." next to your name, they smell blood, and they want to eat your savings accounts. Don't jump in the water with those sharks!

3. Debt-to-Income Ratio

"Most Americans are paying their mortgages on time and are not at risk of foreclosure. But high rates of delinquency and foreclosure can have substantial spillover effects on the housing market, the financial markets, and the broader economy... doing what we can to avoid to prevent foreclosures is not just in the interest of lenders and borrowers. It's in everybody's interest."

— Ben Bernanke (2009)

Do You Know Your Debt-to-Income Ratio?

Due to recent housing price declines, lenders want to see more assets and cash, and they require higher down payments and detailed financial documents to assess your risk as a borrower. They also use your FICO or credit scores.

Lenders learned how much risk was profitable, and one of

Debt-to-Income Ratio

their key tools for assessing a borrower's ability to pay back a loan is debt-to-income (DTI) ratio. Using this banker's tool, we can assess our own risks when buying a home, refinancing, buying a second home, or planning to take on any new debts.

Bankers commonly use two debt-to-income ratios: the top number is called the "housing ratio," and the bottom number is called the "debt-to-income ratio." The top number and the bottom number together are often called "qualifying ratios."

A standard qualifying ratio is written as "28/36." The broker calculates your monthly pre-tax income and multiplies it by 0.28, which is the amount you can reasonably pay toward housing. Then the broker multiplies your pre-tax monthly income by 0.36, which is the amount you can reasonably pay in monthly debt toward housing plus credit cards, car payments, student loans, etc.

To help you calculate your housing and debt-to-income ratio and to see if you're spending a "safe" amount on a mortgage, calculate the following:

Housing Ratio – Determine your top number (also known as the top ratio, the front-end ratio, or PITI)
Add: Mortgage principle + interest + property taxes + homeowner's insurance (often abbreviated PITI)

Debt Ratio – Determine your bottom number (also known as the back-end ratio). PITI + all monthly recurring debt, including credit cards, car loans, student loans, and other recurring debt obligations like child support and alimony

Maximum Housing Ratio – Monthly income x 0.28 = PITI (principle, interest, property tax, insurance)

Maximum Debt Ratio – Monthly income x 0.36 = PITI + all payments on all recurring debt

The housing ratio (top number) was 25 in the 1950s, and bankers calculated no maximum debt ratio. As credit debt grew in the 1970s, lenders added the denominator, the debt ratio. The Federal Housing Authority (FHA), which often takes on higher-risk borrowers, uses a ratio of 29/41. One broker I knew used 33/38, and some lenders allow a maximum debt ratio up to 55.

Years of empiric data allowed lenders to manage risks with profitability. The lower the ratios, the greater the borrower's ability to make monthly payments.

Unfortunately, lenders use these ratios on adjustable-rate mortgages, some of which adjust in three or five years. If a variable mortgage adjusts up, then the debt-to-income ratio adjusts up, too. A borrower who can't make their payments may try to refinance, but if the house depreciates in value and they have less than 20% equity, they may have to pay down the mortgage to refinance at a lower rate. If they initially borrowed with higher housing and debt-to-income ratios, they might not be able to save and pay it down. That's often what prompts foreclosure.

Sadly, many lenders loaned to people with already high monthly debt, and when their mortgages adjusted up, many people couldn't refinance. Foreclosures spread like an epidemic.

So do you know your housing and debt-to-income ratios? Your lender does.

Debt-to-Income Ratio

Calculating Debt-to-Income Ratio

A conventional ratio for a thirty-year fixed loan with a 20% down payment is 28/36.

> **Maximum Housing Ratio = Income x 0.28** – A lender will calculate what you can comfortably afford. If your income is $100,000 a year, they will multiply it by 0.28 to arrive at the top number. So $28,000 is the maximum the lender figures you can spend on principle, interest, taxes, and insurance for a home loan. Divide $28,000 by 12, and the bank figures that you can afford to pay $2,333 a month in housing expenses.
>
> **Top Number = Yearly Pretax Income x 0.28** – This number should be greater than PITI (principle, interest, property taxes, insurance) on the home loan.
>
> **Maximum Debt Ratio = Income x 0.36** – $100,000 x 0.36 = $36,000 per year or $3,000 per month. This is also called the bottom ratio, and it includes the top ratio plus all other recurring monthly expenses, including credit cards, car loans, student loans, and any other recurring debt obligations.

In the above example, a bank would consider a loan if the monthly payment were $2,333 or less and total monthly debts were less than $3,000.

4. Beating the Market

"The best way to measure your investing success is not by whether you are beating the market but by whether you put in place a financial plan and a behavior discipline that are likely to get you where you want to go."

— Benjamin Graham

As investors, we trust our mutual fund managers because they are professionals and we believe they can "beat the market." Market returns are measured by three major market indexes that professional and educated investors follow. These indexes are the Dow Jones Industrial average (often call the "Dow"), the Standard and Poor's 500 (often abbreviated as the "S&P 500"), and the Nasdaq. As of this writing, both the S&P 500 and the Nasdaq dropped 40%, and so did most professionally "managed" mutual funds. So much for paying them to watch your money. They didn't beat the market. Research on mutual fund

Beating the Market

managers shows that they don't beat the market 67% of the time. That's a lousy average. Only one in three mutual fund managers do better than the market index averages.

The best way to avoid that mess is to manage your money yourself. Although mutual fund managers mean well, they often have so much money that they can't get it out when they want to sell. Think about it: if *everyone* wants to sell, a $500 order is easier to fill than an order for $5 million. If the market is full of sellers but has no buyers, larger investors and mutual funds can get hurt.

Bill Miller is an all-star investor whose mutual fund beat the S&P 500 twelve years in a row. His fund owned 20% of Amazon's stock, and when it went up, his fund did well. But when he wanted to sell to lock in profits, there were no more buyers for his millions of Amazon shares. You and I can dart in and out because we have small stock orders and can often sell the same day, and often we can sell within minutes by going to a website, punching in a few numbers, and placing a sell order.

I know many of you sold stocks because the market continued to decline. I heard more than one person say, "My 401k is now a 201k." Anyone who held on to their stocks in this recent stock market downturn lost significant portions of their retirement accounts.

If you did sell and you're sitting on cash, waiting for the market to rebound, here's something to think about when you reenter the market: the mutual funds want you to ride the market down and not sell. If you didn't listen to them and cashed out, consider some new exchange traded funds (ETFs), which are mutual funds that trade like a stock. Brokers charge you to buy and sell an ETF just like a stock.

Investment Guide for Doctors

Bull Market ETFs

These ETFs move three times the market indexes:

TNA — 3x small cap bull
TQQQ — 3x Nasdaq bull
SPXL — 3x S&P 500
UDOW — 3x Dow
FAS — 3x financial bull

These ETFs move twice the market indexes:

QLD — 2x Nasdaq
SSO — 2x S&P 500
DDM — 2x Dow

These ETFs move one time the market indexes:

SPY — 1X S&P 500
QQQ — 1x Nasdaq
DIA — 1x Dow

Pyramiding: A Market Reentry Strategy

If you have a lot of cash, you may want to consider a re-entry strategy. Allocate the funds you want to invest, then pick a few of the above indexes.

Say you want to invest $5,000 in an ETF. Divide $5,000 into these investment allocations: 1/6, 1/6, 1/3, and 1/3. In cash terms it looks like this: $833, $833, $1,667, and $1,667. Your first purchase of the stock or the ETF should be $833.

Beating the Market

Be sure to use a stop loss if your stock goes below 10% (I use 7% to 8% if I can catch it). If you "stop out" to protect capital at 10%, you lose about $84. If you put the whole $5,000 in at once and "stopped out," you would lose $500, which is a lot more than $84. But if you add the second 1/6 after your first 1/6 makes a 2% to 3% gain, you have insurance now and are in for 1/3 of your investment. Then if it goes up 2% to 3% again, you can add the second 1/3, then another 2% to 3% for the last 1/3. This strategy of investing is sometimes called pyramiding because it involves adding funds in steps as the stock goes up.

Each small gain insures your next purchase to a certain extent, assuming you keep a stop loss. Unless you think the market will go down, then you can invest in ETF bear funds that go up when the market goes down. BGZ is a former exchange-traded funded that goes down three times as fast as the large caps. I didn't include bear market funds because, in general, it's much more difficult to short the market (make money when the stock market declines) than it is to make money when the stock market is rising.

I hope you don't make the mistake, as I did, of thinking that there will be a big pull back in financials right before they skyrocketed forward. I once invested in SKF, a financial bear fund ETF that rises when the financials go down. It rises twice as fast as the financial index goes down. I purchased the SKF shares and placed a stop loss order to sell, if my ETF went down below 8% of my purchase price. A few days after my purchase, SKF dropped 18% in one day! Financial stocks were rallying, but I bet they would drop.

My stop loss (an order to sell) got passed over, and SKF wasn't sold as I had requested at an 8% loss. There were too many people trying to sell, and the brokerage firm didn't fill my sell order. I eventually sold, but the value was lower than my 8% stop loss. I sold at an 18% loss! Some people might think it was hopeless and leave the money in until it comes back up. No way! I sold on the next day's open, and over the next few days, SKF declined 33% below my initial purchase. The stop loss order was not effective insurance.

Unless you haven't been listening to the news, Uncle Sam will not let the banks fail. Now I see there can be no safer investment with that type of government support. Forget the long-term consequences of government regulations on the economy. The market uptrends before an economic recovery, and job growth occurs after businesses become profitable and look to expand. Let's hope Bob Brinker, *Investor Business Daily*, and VectorVest are correct and the market continues to rise.

5. Predicting Stock Market Direction

"Predictions about the direction of the stock market tell you nothing about where stocks are headed, but a whole lot about the person doing the predicting."

— Warren Buffett

In the book *The Next Great Bubble Boom*, Harry S. Dent predicted that the Dow would hit new highs in early 2006 but would crash in 2010 to 2012. Bob Brinker predicts the market is headed up within the next several months. Careful though, usually there is a pull back before most rallies. Both of these individuals who try to time the market use their own proprietary models to help them predict stock market direction. How can you, the individual investor, learn to predict market direction yourself?

Predicting market direction is critical to investing. "Buy and hold" investors lost 60% in the Nasdaq market during the tech bubble, starting in March of 2000 and continuing until March of

Predicting Stock Market Direction

2003. Buy-and-hold was 401k and retirement investment suicide! A 50% loss requires a 100% investment return to get back to even. It's better to not make money and to hold cash than to invest and lose money. Both Dent and Brinker made correct buy-and-sell recommendations during the tech bubble.

Technical analysis is like reading x-rays or blood tests. It allows you to analyze stocks by looking at their charts, and it can help individual investors understand the health of market trends and individual stocks. *High Probability Trading* by Marcel Lind can teach you to interpret easily produced technical charts on Yahoo Finance. Some of the world's greatest traders use trend following models... yes, they use only charts and graphs! Interestingly, these technical indicators all say that the market trend is likely higher in the near future. I suggest starting with slow stochastics, relative strength, and MACD. Understanding these will improve your ability to predict market direction. But these indicators have limits, of course, because there's no absolute certain investment. Nothing in investing is fool-proof, especially "buy and hold!"

I believe that some people can predict general stock market direction. Bob Brinker, the author of *Market Timer*, a subscription newsletter, has been doing it for twenty years. But the truth is that no human or computer program can predict the direction of the stock market with 100% accuracy. That said, an individual investor can likely outperform two-thirds of all managed mutual funds, if you simply buy an S&P 500 or Nasdaq exchange traded fund or a mutual fund that follows these indexes.

6. Index Investing

"Most institutional and individual investors will find the best way to own common stock is through an index fund that charges minimal fees. Those following this path are sure to beat the net results delivered by the great majority of investment professionals."

— Warren Buffet

An index fund is a mutual fund or an exchange traded fund that attempts to match the performance of a market index. The most common stock market index matches the S&P 500, which is a composite of America's largest 500 companies. In our Fidelity 401k plan, BGI Equity is the only index fund, and it's indexed with the S&P 500. Unfortunately, it will close to new investors and to Kaiser physician investors through our 401k plans at the end of July.

Index Investing

Another way to invest in an index fund is to purchase exchange traded funds (ETFs). You can do that by signing up for a brokerage link account. Just call Fidelity and ask them. It will cost $50 a year, but it's well worth the ability to buy and sell both ETFs and individual stocks (buying individual stocks is the reason that investing is so risky).

There are many ETFs that also follow the stock market indexes. For example, SPYDER (symbol SPY) is an ETF that attempts to match the performance of the S&P 500. The most popular ETF index is the Cubes (symbol QQQ), which attempts to match the performance of the Nasdaq 100 index. The Cubes are heavily loaded with technology stocks. DIAMONDS (symbol DIA) is another ETF, and it tracts the Dow Jones Industrial average, which is composed of thirty common stocks.

An ETF is like buying a stock as they are bought and sold throughout the day, whereas a mutual fund can only be bought at the end of the day. I've included some advantages and disadvantages of exchange-traded funds below.

Common Exchange Traded Funds (ETFs)

Symbol
QQQ – Cubes tracks the Nasdaq 100
DIA – DIAMONDS tracks the Dow
SPY – SPYDER tracks the S&P 500

Advantages of ETFs

ETFs are inexpensive, and you can track the price of the fund throughout the day. There's no 2% selling penalty if you sell before owning it two months, which is what most mutual funds charge. You can also buy an ETF on margin, and you can buy and trade throughout the day. It's a great way to diversify.

Disadvantages of ETFs

You will pay a trading fee to buy and sell ETFs, just like a stock. The ETF may trade above or below the index or underly holding it's tracking. One major disadvantage of ETF index funds is that it would be expensive to dollar-cost average into an ETF every month or bimonthly because each time you make a new purchase, you incur a charge.

Dollar-cost averaging involves buying more shares when a stock, ETF, or mutual fund drops and fewer shares when the value increases. Dollar-cost averaging decreases the risk of putting all your investment in at the high point of the market and watching it go straight down. But it also decreases your chance of getting in on the ground floor and hitting a homerun.

Dollar-cost averaging into an index mutual fund with direct withdrawals into a 401k plan from one's regular paycheck is sound advice for most investors, especially if those funds are directed into an index fund that matches the returns of the S&P 500.

So what do Nobel Prize economists say about index funds? Michael Jenson won the 1965 Nobel Prize for a study that showed that only 26 out of 115 actively managed funds from 1945 to 1965 outperformed the market. In 1975, John Bogle helped develop the first index fund available to private investors. The fund was eventually called the Vanguard 500, which followed the S&P 500. This fund surpassed the $100

Index Investing

billion assets milestone in 1999, and now it has more assets than the famous Magellan Fund, which Peter Lynch once ran. Bogle's thesis was entitled "Mutual Funds Cannot Make Claims of Superiority Over the Market Averages."

7. The Great Recession

"Live for now, but plan for the future. You just might get it."

— A wise, retired ninety-year-old wine maker

The Recession and Investing for 2009

Investing in Harsh Economic Times

Many people lost investing confidence early in our present economic recession. Wall Street corruption eroded investors 401k savings. Thousands of people lost hard earned retirement nest eggs in Bernie Madoff's $50 billion Ponzi scheme. One doctor lost $5 million dollars to Madoff, and at seventy-five years old, he couldn't afford to retire! CNN reports that "mini Madoffs" are stealing investors' money all over the country.

The housing bubble burst, then foreclosures exploded in 2008. According to Fox News, more than two million homes

The Great Recession

were foreclosed last year. Yahoo posted more than 4,000 foreclosures in San Jose in January of 2009. Bay Area home prices dropped 20% in some areas, vaporizing our home equity. California Realtors and contractors now seek jobs, and state unemployment rises over 7%.

US stock market indexes plummeted 40% in 2008, dragging down most of our 401k retirement funds in the wake of Wall Street's "deleveraging." Even President Barack Obama said that it's "shameful" that bank executives earned $20 billion in bonuses as they ran their companies into insolvency. Now taxpayers support banks and car companies on the brink of bankruptcy.

With this torrent of investing mayhem, is it even worth saving and investing in 2009? Here are three suggestions for investing in these harsh economic times:

1. **Keep Contributing to Your 401k** – Our 401k plans allow us to save up to $20,500 in 2022. You can add the "catch up" of $6,000 in 2022 if you're over 50. Because 401k funds go directly into your account before taxes, you essentially make at least 35% on your money, depending on your tax bracket. You can begin tapping into it at 59½ without paying the 10% withdrawal penalty, and you don't pay taxes until you withdraw from it. Where else can you get that type of return? If you've got a source, let me know. My guess is their nose is as long as Pinocchio, and they are ripping people off like Madoff. Even if you're out of the market and gradually getting back in, adding to your 401k makes a lot of sense. As long as you're a long-term investor.

2. **Pay Down Your Mortgage** – Paying down mortgage debt may lower your retirement age. It's a low-risk investment. Consider adding small monthly principal payments. Add an additional principal payment each month, and you can pay of the loan in half the time. Figure interest savings with online calculators at Yahoo Financial.

A home mortgage is second only to taxes as life's greatest expense.

3. **Make a Retirement Plan** – At age 59½, we're eligible to start taking out of our 401k and IRA without the 10% withdrawal penalty. At 62, many become eligible for partial Social Security retirement benefits. Full Social Security benefits occur at your official retirement age. Presently, if you're born after 1960, your retirement age is 67. How much do you plan to save in your nest egg? And at what age will you start to take distributions. How about your pension? Do you plan to work part time in retirement? I know one local retired physician who works in the community, and I know another working as a locum tenens, and he enjoys the adventures. I'm sure the money doesn't hurt.

Try these online retirement calculators:

- Kaiser's retirement planning website: www.tpmgplanner.com

The Great Recession

- Yahoo.com – User-friendly home mortgage and retirement calculators
- 401k.com – Fidelity's educational center for retirement planning
- SSA.com – Social Security helps figure retirement benefits

Caution: the quality of calculators varies, and many make you assume yearly investment returns and inflation. Many financial advisors use 6% to 7% yearly returns and 3% inflation as a "guestimate." But don't let any advisor fool you, NO ONE knows exactly what those numbers will be, and there are no sure-thing investments. Some of our retirement calculations will fall short, especially if monthly expenses exceed monthly income. In USA Today's book *Retire Happy*, the authors state that many people over-invest in their retirement and live pretty comfortably.

I really like my friend's father's investment advice: "Live for today, but plan for tomorrow. You just might get it." Can't beat that with a bailout!

Current Income Sources During Retirement:

Social Security — 39%
Employment — 26%
Pensions — 19%
Savings and Investments — 16%

8. Is Your Money Safe?

"A penny saved is a penny earned."

— Benjamin Franklin

"The safe way to double your money is to fold it over once and put it in your pocket."

— Kin Hubbard

Are our retirement funds safe? Bear Stearns was a publicly traded company that offered retirement, investment, and college savings advisory services, but they became insolvent in 2008. Their shares went from $140 to $2. Oh, the irony of financial advisors going bankrupt! Investors at Bear Stearns lost money, employees lost their jobs, and some went to jail.

What if Fidelity goes bankrupt? Don't think it could happen?

Is Your Money Safe?

Study financial and banking stocks on Yahoo, but don't do it before going to bed. It could cause insomnia.

I called Fidelity and looked on their website, www.fidelity.com. Fortunately, Fidelity does carry investor insurance with the Securities Investors Protection Corporation (SIPC), which insures our accounts up to $500,000, including $100,000 in cash. Additional "unlimited protection" is covered under the Customer Asset Protection Company (CAPCO). But don't take my word for it. Go to www.sipc.com and www.fidelity.com to learn more.

How Safe Is Your Checking and Savings Account?

The Federal Deposit Insurance Corporation (FDIC) recently declared that the number of banks on its unnamed "troubled list" increased from 90 to 117. They obviously didn't name those banks, otherwise people would make runs on them like they did on Indymac Bank in Southern California. In July, depositors arrived early before Indymac's doors opened, hoping that enough money was left in the bank to get their hard-earned savings out.

People lost savings above the $100,000 insured by the FDIC, but they could have avoided any loss by transferring money above the FDIC insured $100,000 into another FDIC-insured bank. If you have this problem, lucky you! Making sure that all your savings are FDIC insured will cure the insomnia triggered by your study of financial and banking stocks on Yahoo.

The FDIC insures checking and savings up to $100,000 if a bank becomes insolvent or bankrupt. Does your bank have FDIC insurance? Keep in mind that you could lose money above that amount, even with insurance, if your bank becomes insolvent.

There's no reason to keep more than $100,000 in a single bank. If you have a joint account with your spouse, it may be insured up to $200,000. Additionally, you can have an individual account insured up to $100,000—and you may have an IRA that is protected up to $250,000. Unlike the value in your house, you can have FDIC insurance on your cash savings accounts. But don't take my word for it. Enter your bank's name on the website www.fdic.com and see if your bank is FDIC insured. If not, get your cash into an FDIC-insured bank. I checked two large banks—Wells Fargo and Bank of America—and both have full FDIC insurance.

About fifteen years ago, after studying and preparing for months, I invested in my first mutual fund. I saved diligently to put $1,200 in an American Century fund and saw it plummet to $700 in six months. And that, of course, was my fault. But if it was in cash at a FDIC-insured bank or an SIPC-insured investment house (or even better, CAPCO), I wouldn't have lost a dime, and at no risk.

Said simply, check your banks. Is your money safe?

9. The 1% Home Loan

Buying real estate can be a sound investment, and you can always live in a house. It's also a way to diversify so you don't lose the money you put into real estate when the stock market drops.

Some quacks live to make a buck from you. Be forewarned that if a loan broker asks, "What do you do for a living?" and you respond, "I'm a doctor," you're essentially putting a big green sign on your forehead that says, "SUCKER." To some loan agents, the "S" will look like a dollar sign.

I once met "Eric the Refrigerator," a loan broker from World Financial Group, who offered a 1% payment loan. A real estate agent I didn't know and met only once while looking at an open house in my neighborhood referred me to him. Eric had recently graduated from San Jose State. He'd majored in football, and he certainly saw the "SUCKER" sign on my forehead. The dollar signs sprouted green wings and flew about my head. This loan, a negative amortization loan, isn't easy to understand, and he couldn't explain it to me. I don't believe he even understood it himself.

I could decrease my monthly mortgage payment from $2,500 a month to $1,250 a month, but the interest rate was variable, starting at 5%. Each month my statement gave three options: the 1% payment, the interest-only payment (with a current variable rate of 5%), or interest payment with an amortization of the principle. The problem with a 1% payment is that any interest difference between the recent 5% variable rate and the 1% is added to your home's principle. Sound confusing? That's because it is, and that's why Eric couldn't explain it.

So I visited another loan agent in Fremont, referred by a friend. He said that he had taken an entire course on the "neg-am" loan. In a nutshell, he said, "You owe more on your home loan with the 1% payment option." The dollar signs with wings were fanning the sweat off my forehead.

Eric and I set a time for me to sign the loan at my house Friday after work. That day I was at work in a meeting that ran late, so I called him on his cell phone, figuring he was waiting in the driveway for me. He responded, "I'm at my office" and promptly put me on hold. He came back in ten minutes and said, "Can I call you right back?" He paged me fifteen minutes later. When I called him back, the line was busy. My meeting finished, I went home and called Eric several more times. His line was always busy. Eric didn't call again until Monday morning, when he asked, "Can we set a time to sign the loan papers?" HELLO!

It got worse. To get the loan, I had to give him my credit card number to pay for a credit check. The credit check is negotiable, and lenders typically pay this for you. It might be the case that loan agents want you to pay for the credit check if they see the

"SUCKER" sign on your forehead. I paid for the credit check, and he charged $100 for a security check so I could get on a pyramid scheme with him. But I didn't authorize the charge and didn't want any part of the scheme. By this time, the winged dollar signs had completely dried the sweat on my face. The guy had stolen $100 from my credit card!

And he wasn't finished yet. Eric claimed that he sold investments at the World Financial Group, and he had a life insurance policy that paid a guaranteed 12% per year. Eric brought in some young kid from Chicago, who explained a life insurance annuity. The annuity was two years old, and the kid couldn't give me a track record of the investment management team. A kid from Chicago was selling me an annuity and Eric the Refrigerator was selling a negative amortization loan, and I believe it was then that I saw the chiming dollar signs coming from both their eye sockets.

But then things got better. I didn't get a loan with Eric the Refrigerator. Nor did I purchase an annuity with the kid from Chicago. I called my previous loan agent. I trusted her, and she explained the neg-am loan and said it was a viable option. "I can get you one of those if you want, but you will owe more on your house when you go to sell it." Essentially you pay the monthly interest with the equity in your home. The bank makes you pay either way, in cash or in home equity.

I learned a valuable lesson, and I clearly understand the world better. I now know that if you buy or refinance your house, you should ask these questions: Are the loan agents trustworthy? Were they referred from a colleague or family who had good experiences with them? Do they pass the "sniff test," or does something smell fishy? Zig Ziggler said, "You can't make a good deal with a bad person." You can't do business with

The 1% Home Loan

crooks, charlatans, or people with green dollar signs flashing in their eye sockets. The eyes are just reflecting what they see on your forehead. If you feel the sweat being fanned on your forehead when you're looking for a cheap home loan, it could be that the green dollar signs have sprouted wings.

10. Playing Defense

"The first rule of investing is to not lose money. The second rule is to never forget rule number one."

— Warrant Buffet

The Case for Cowardice

It's scary looking at our retirement accounts, especially for the buy-and-hold investor. But some say, "Don't worry. The market will come back." Since the stock market's peak in 2000, it hasn't come back, and in recent months, the market is more than 15% off its high. In 2000, the Nasdaq was about 4,000, and today, eight years later, it's roughly 2,300.

Recently, I was heavily margined in my cash account, meaning that I had borrowed money to invest. It was glorious, I was up 30% last year and 20% the year before. Bob Brinker, my investment guru, said to get in the market when the S&P 500

Playing Defense

was under 1,450. I thought this was my chance, I got fully margined (borrowed and leveraged as much as I could) under 1,450. In his last six recommendations, the market always shot up, and he was predicting a rise to 1,600. But in this, his seventh prediction, the market didn't turn up as he had predicted. As of this writing, it's at 1,280, a 12% drop.

I have set up cowardly rules for my own investing, and with true humility and ignorance, I decided not to follow them. Inside my head, I heard an echo… *Don't worry… The market will come back.* And besides, who am I to go against Bob Brinker, who recommend to get out of the stock market before the great tech bubble in 2000?

Passively, I was in the QLD, an exchange traded fund (ETF) that doubles the Nasdaq market. If the Nasdaq goes up 1%, this ETF goes up 2%. And if the market goes down 1%, you lose 2%. BUT I WAS ON MARGIN. So if the market went up 1%, I was up 4%. And if the market went down 1%, my account dropped 4%. This is called leveraged investing. So, I passively watched my account go past my rule, which states:

Sell any investments that go below 7% of purchase price.

But worse, I didn't follow my margin rule:

When on margin, if your account loses 2% to 3% in a week, sell and get off margin.

A loss of 2% to 3% means that you're hedged in the wrong direction. In the words of environmentalist Steve Irwin, this spells, "Danger, danger, danger!" But I kept telling myself, *Don't worry. The market will come back.*

The pain mounted, and I was off 15% on this investment. I had hedged for a large loss, and I stopped thinking, *Don't worry. The market will come back.* I began thinking, *How much do I have left?*

I sold way below where I usually would have... Who am I to go against Bob Brinker? He was wrong, and the rule was right, as it always has been. So I sold at a loss, and the market went down another 12%. If I had held to that point, it would have meant another 25% loss! I'm now sitting on cash, watching the market continue to drop. And I'm mad at myself for trusting my investment guru Bob Brinker and for not following Warren Buffet's first rule of investing. Yes, the cowardly don't-lose-money rule.

Of course, the more important investing rule is to not lose your nest egg! Markets don't always come back, as recent history has shown. Some say that the stock market always comes back, but sometimes that can take years. After the tech bubble of 2000, it actually took thirteen years for the Nasdaq to recover.

Investor's Business Daily noted in April of 2022, "The last time the economy was in a long-term inflationary period was in 1968 to 1982. The S&P 500 closed at 108.37 in November 1968. At the end of July 1982, it stood at 107.09. Over nearly 14 years that works out to a total loss of 1.2%."

11. Fundamentals of Asset Allocation

"Asset allocation is an investment strategy that attempts to balance risk versus reward by adjusting the percentage of each asset in an entire portfolio according to the investor's risk tolerance, goals, and investment time frame."

— Wikipedia

Asset allocation is important to any investor because it helps you manage investment risks. Several studies have shown that it's the most important factor controlling investment risks and returns. Your entire portfolio is 100% of your investment assets, and the two most common asset classes are stocks and bonds.

The longer you have until retirement, the more risk you can take investing in stocks. If you have more than ten years to retire, a good allocation is 70% in funds that track the S&P 500, 10% in international stocks, 10% in small caps, and 10% in individual stocks. This asset allocation is considered aggressive because it's all in stocks and no bonds.

Historically, index funds outperform two-thirds of all professionally managed mutual funds. Allocating the majority of assets with a group of stocks using index funds like the Wilshire 5000 or S&P 500 decreases overall investment risks. Individual stocks carry a much higher risk.

As we approach or enter retirement, we want to decrease our stock investment risk and preserve capital. Most people consider allocating a large portion of their portfolio in bonds or fixed income investments like certificates of deposit as they approach or are in retirement. This allows you to preserve capital, and it can provide interest from investments to use for living expenses. An example asset allocation in retirement is 70% bonds, 20% treasuries, and 10% in broad market indexes.

Investing involves time, risks, and rewards. Asset allocation is a great tool to help control risks over time and increase your potential rewards.

12. Mad Money: Picking Individual Stocks

"After a lifetime of picking stocks, I have to admit that Bogle's arguments in favor of the index fund have me thinking of joining him rather than trying to beat him."

— Jim Cramer, host of the TV show *Mad Money*

Knowing when to buy individual stocks is as much an art as knowing when to sell. Jim Cramer, host of CNN's *Mad Money*, advises to, "Buy and homework. Not buy and hold."

The two most important factors in picking a good stock are earnings and growth. Be careful! You must follow both the company and the stock. Microsoft has tremendous earnings, but its stock hasn't moved in the last four years. If you can't follow the company and its stock on a regular—preferable daily—basis, then don't buy individual stocks.

To find quality stocks, consider *Investor's Business Daily*, an

Mad Money: Picking Individual Stocks

investment newspaper available at some bookstores, magazine stands, and online. The Monday issue profiles "The IBD 100," offering detailed graphs and stock buying points. They use and teach technical analysis, which is basically following graphs. If you see a company you like, then go to Google—which is a great stock, in my opinion—or Yahoo and research the company more. Make sure you think the company has positive earnings and growth.

Limiting your individual stock exposure is critical in a long-term investment plan. Bob Brinker, the host of the investing radio show *Money Talk* (KGO 810 AM radio), suggests that you invest no more than 4% of your total portfolio in any one stock. Jim Cramer recommends up to 20% of your *Mad Money* disposable income for speculative stocks. Personally, I have lost 50% overnight on one stock, one that was recommended by the investing company VectorVest. No one, I believe, has ever seen the entire stock market lose 50% in one day. Individual stocks on the other hand, have a higher chance of steep declines, and some stocks disappear altogether after their company goes bankrupt.

Investor's Business Daily recommends selling any stock that loses 8% or more from your purchase price. If you sell stocks that gain 20% or more, you can lose twice and win once and come out ahead.

You can never get hurt selling a stock at a profit. I have friends and family that have come out of retirement and lost fortunes because they watched a stock go up, and then they watched their stock go down. They never sold for a profit. Yes, you may lose some profits by selling, but you decrease your risk once you sell to lock in gains.

These guidelines—along with luck and a bull market—could

make you rich. But then again, who really has time for all the homework required for individual stocks. One way out is to watch Jim Cramer's *Mad Money* on CNN. He does the homework for you. He's nuts, but he's entertaining, and he's a stock-picking genius who loves telling you about his homework.

13. Getting Whipsawed

"Whipsaw describes the movement of a stock when, at a particular time, the security's price is moving in one direction but then quickly pivots to move in the opposite direction. There are two types of whipsaw patterns. The first involves an upward movement in a share price, which is then followed by a drastic downward move causing the share's price to fall relative to its original position. The second type occurs when a share price drops in value for a short time and then suddenly surges upward to a positive gain relative to the stock's original position."

— Investopedia

The market's recent upturn follows a mid-presidential year correction of about 10%. The Dow is at near all-time highs after recovering from the 2000 tech bubble, and it's performing better than the Nasdaq and the S&P 500.

Getting Whipsawed

I previously purchased Hanson (symbol HAN) and accumulated shares a few at a time, increasing my holding from $92 to $102. The stock ran up to $200 in three months, with hardly a day of hard selling on high volume. Around May 11, Hanson ran up 14% a day for two days. That's 28% in two days! After that climax run, I sold all my shares at $185, on the first day of heavy distribution. That was a profit of 85%.

My portfolio was up 20% for the year, and it was only March! I have held cash since, as I slowly sold off both my losers and winners as they met heavy volume distribution days. I sold all my stocks and was out of the market until about a month ago.

The general market trend as of this writing is back in the positive direction. Recently, I staked a position in GROW, an investment company that a colleague who works in urgent care introduced me to. I accumulated GROW stock, and after several pyramiding buys (buying more as it goes up), the stock blasted up 30% in about two weeks. Owning 3,000 shares, I was up 15% in two weeks. I added an additional 2,000. Even with the added shares, I was up 5%. I thought, *Here's another Hanson*, where I nearly doubled my investment. Then the uptrend in the stock stopped abruptly, and it saw two heavy days of distribution. I was down 5% in one day. The next day, the stock dropped another 12%. It was the highest one-day, single-stock loss in my entire investment experience.

I got whipsawed, which is buying on an uptrend and getting shaken out because of a quick downturn in the stock price. Unlike Hanson, which I purchased before the climax run, I bought GROW during its end-stage climax run, which is a common way for a good stock to end its upswing.

I also got whipsawed with Chicago Mercantile Exchange

(CME), a financial services company. It was up 30% in two weeks, and then as it dove down, I sold at the market for a 4% total gain. I hear of many investors getting whipsawed. Bob Brinker and Jim Cramer both think that the market will rise by year's end, but no one really knows. It may sell off as fast as the tech bubble in 2000, after the Nasdaq market doubled from October of 1999 to March of 2000. The last stages of a market cycle are when it really accelerates before the collapse.

The best investors always sell on the way up. Bob Brinker's sell sign came in January of 2000. The market topped in March. It was an extraordinary climax run, especially in tech stocks, where mania took over and where no sensible valuation exists. Price-to-earnings ratios were at extreme levels, expanding the great boom to climax in March of 2000. If you sold into the mania, you banked a tidy profit. The problem, of course, was that not many sold. I sold only because I trusted Bob Brinker 100%, and I had already made a good profit.

The luckiest stock investment that I owned was Intel, which I bought at $22 and again at $25. Intel rose to $110—a "double double!" The Bob Brinker sell signal came March 11, 2003, but the stock market continued to rise rapidly for a while. He began getting death threats after telling people to sell their stocks and mutual fund holdings. I went entirely into cash, as he had recommended, and I didn't make much in a money market account. More importantly, I wasn't going to lose money if the market took a downturn, as Brinker predicted.

After I sold and put everything I had into a money market account, Intel zoomed up to a peak of around $155. I missed another 30% gain, but no one can predict the bottom or the top. Those who bought late into the market, into this climax run, all

Getting Whipsawed

lost money. By March of 2021, the stock market had begun its sharp decline, giving back the gains it produced in the previous six months. Getting whipsawed isn't a pleasant experience, but it's one that most who invest will experience—and remember.

14. Margin Management: Using Leverage

Investing on margin means borrowing money from your broker to use for investments.

When to Get on Margin

Only go on margin or use borrowed money when the market is clearly in an uptrend and you're winning, making some profits on your investments. During a bull run, many stocks break out over several months. In an uptrend, it's better to gradually go on margin as you're winning. For example, if your portfolio goes up 2% to 3% for a few weeks and there's a broad market rally, it could be a good idea to go on margin.

It might be best to use margin only on follow-up buys, after you have profited from your initial purchase of a stock. A second purchase is only added when you already have a gain on your initial purchase. The initial gain can be used as insurance. Adding to a stock position as it goes up is called pyramiding.

Margin Management: Using Leverage

Consider adding margin funds only when you're winning (i.e., 1% to 2% a week for a few weeks).

When to Get off Margin

Get off margin if your stocks are losing or if your portfolio loses more than 2% to 3% in one week. If you need to sell more than two stocks in a week because they lose 7% to 8%, consider getting off margin. Get off margin and raise cash when the MARKET REVERSES from an uptrend to a downtrend. Get off margin when you aren't sure of the market's direction.

Beginning investors shouldn't use margin until after three to five years of investing experience. Remember that you lose twice as fast when you're on margin.

A 7% loss on margin takes a 15% gain to get back to zero!

A 50% loss takes a 100% gain to get back to zero, even if you aren't on margin.

You Must First Minimize Losses

You win twice as big on margin, but the losses are also twice as big. Leverage works both ways. Margin is like wetting the sails of a boat. You move faster with the wind, but in a storm, it's better to have your sails down. When the market starts to decline, get off margin. Intelligently used, it's an excellent tool, but it can hurt if you aren't paying attention to your portfolio. If you can't watch your account, don't be on margin.

Getting Back a Loss Is More Difficult on Margin

It's not good to use borrowed money for an initial stock purchase, only on follow-up buys. Margin investments are best for second positions. The fact that the first one went up and you're adding to it confirms that your stock is in bull mode.

Since three of every four stocks follow the general market direction, if you're adding shares to a stock you purchased as it went up, you're likely going up with the market. But if you get a few sudden declines on several stocks that you purchased as prices rose, sell some of the stock, especially if the entire stock market is in a sudden decline. You can buy the shares back if the market rebounds.

Buy and sell your initial stock purchases off margin, even if you think you have a very strong stock. If it's early in a market rally, you may have moved too soon, and you may get shaken out early. For example, I bought Hanson stock too soon. Then I bought and sold it repeatedly, until it took off upward. Then I let it ride for an 85% gain. (Note: usually I get shaken out of a stock more often than one takes off.) If I had bought and sold shares of GROW, then even though I got shaken out, if I had stuck with it and purchased shares as it had gone up again, I would have potentially had the huge double in gains I was expecting! I nailed the stock, but I gave up on it too soon. GROW did double, but I was whipsawed out before it did.

It's okay to buy in and out. This is the individual investors advantage over large institutional investors. Most large mutual funds purchase stocks over several days or weeks, typically at different prices. It takes time for their orders to get filled because they have huge amounts of stock to purchase. The individual investor has a smaller number of shares than the mutual funds,

Margin Management: Using Leverage

which makes it easier and faster for the individual to buy and sell their stock positions.

Times to Get off Margin

- When your account loses 2% to 3% in a week
- If you aren't winning (i.e., you're stopped out 7% to 8% on your last two or three stock picks)
- Don't make initial purchases on margin

Decrease stock and market exposure if you're losing, if the market tops, or if the market is beginning a downward trend.

Consequences of Poor Margin Management

Losing 2% to 3% on an individual stock on margin means that you're losing 4% to 6% of the actual amount shown on your daily account! This means you have to gain about 7% to get it back to zero.

On Margin, a 7% Loss Is Really a 15% Loss!

It's risky to purchase your initial stock positions on margin, unless you see something extraordinary and you're winning all around. Even then, you make *one and only one* exception. The stock and position should be exceptional because if you lose 7% on the second or on a follow-up stock purchase, you're losing 15% of the total position. So if you're on margin, you must sell the second position if it comes back to zero because it retraced the entire gain. You lose a larger amount if you wait until a stop loss of 7%.

It should be fine to hold quality stocks in a strong market that pulls back after its initial run-up. Many strong stocks need some room to breathe. Remember defense first. In a very rocky market, you may want to sell even those stocks not on margin when they lose all their advance. Especially if the market trend is changing.

Remember the sell rule: If a stock is up 8% after a second purchase and your stock drops to zero, get out and call it a draw.

An 8% loss on margin takes a 15% percent gain to get back the money lost.

A 33% decrease needs a 50% increase to get back the lost money.

A 50% loss requires a 100% return to get back your money.

If you're on margin and lose 50%, you may well have lost most everything already because you have to pay the money back that you borrowed from your broker.

Purchasing stocks on margin is very risky business. It's investing with borrowed money, and the money needs to be paid back, even if you lose the borrowed money purchasing stocks. Other ways to leverage include using your home equity line of credit to invest in stocks or mutual funds and purchasing exchange traded funds that double or triple the market averages. These are not leveraged techniques that I recommend for conservative investors, although I have done all of them myself.

The following chart lists the exchange-traded funds that follow the market indexes and the exchange-traded funds that double or triple the market indexes.

Margin Management: Using Leverage

Exchange Traded Funds (ETF) Indexes

Standard Market ETFs

QQQQ — 100% Nasdaq 100
SPY — 100% S&P 500
IWP — 100% Mid cap
DIA — 100% Dow

Leveraged ETFs – 200% of Market Indexes

QLD — 200% Nasdaq
SSO — 200% S&P 500
MVV — 200% Mid cap
DDM — 200% Dow

Leveraged ETFs – 300% of Market Indexes

TNA — 300% Small cap bull
TQQQ — 300% Nasdaq bull
SPXL — 300% S&P 500
UDOW — 300% Dow
FAS — 300% Financial bull

15. A Financial, Personal, and Legacy Retirement Plan

"Age is an issue of mind over matter. If you don't mind, it doesn't matter."

— Mark Twain

"A budget can lead to a surplus of funds to invest in, which overtime can lead to a fortune."

— Brian Buffini

"You know you're getting old when you bend down to tie your shoelaces and wonder what else you could do while down there," George Burns once said. Are you getting older without a retirement plan? Several colleagues have cell phones that count down the years, days, and minutes until retirement. Here are three steps for you to consider. Each has three key ideas. Having

A Financial, Personal, and Legacy Retirement Plan

a balanced financial, personal, and legacy plan could set you up for a happy retirement.

Step 1: Financial Plan

Kaiser Permanente has a three-step approach to help finance our retirements:

Plan 1 – Pension Plan

The pension plan is based on the number of years you work. Each year of the first twenty years of working with the group is 2%, then it's 1% a year for the next ten years. That amount is based on the highest three-year average of salary and bonus compensation.

For example, if your highest average salary over three years while working was $100K and you worked thirty years with the medical group:

$$\$100K/year \times 20 \text{ years } @ 2\% = \$40K$$
$$+ 10 \text{ years } @ 1\% = \$10K$$

If you add the $40K and the $10K, you get $50K per year in retirement pension benefits.

Plan 2 – Kaiser Permanente Contribution Plan

Each month the medical group contributes funds to our retirement plan, specifically into our Fidelity accounts. These funds are 100% vested after five years of service with the group. Be sure you allocate these funds into a mutual fund or an investment of your choosing. I recently reviewed mine and discovered that it was going into a money market cash fund, which is basically a savings account. That's not a good idea given that the S&P 500 stock market went up 30% in 2013.

Plan 3 – 401k Plan

Our 401k plan allows us to make voluntary pre-tax contributions to our chosen retirement investments. The maximum contribution in 2022 is $20,500, with a catch-up contribution—if you're fifty years old or over—of $6,500 for a total of $27,000 (you can check www.irs.gov online because contribution limits change often). Be sure to set up a portion of each paycheck into a 401k, if you haven't already done so. You can adjust the percentage of each paycheck (i.e., 10%) to put into your 401k. You should be aware that you need to direct these funds into an investment of your choice, like a mutual fund.

Step 2: Personal Plan

1. **Make a bucket list** – Make sure you have a list of things you want to do. Many of my patients go back to work after getting pensions because they are young, they get bored, and they want something to do. Write a book, travel, spend time with grandkids—these are common bucket-list items. Sitting around and relaxing may sound good, but after resting for some number of months or years, most retirees want to do things.
2. **Know where you want to live** – According to Richard Stim and Ralph Warner's book *Retire Happy*, "Studies show that the most powerful predictor of life satisfaction after retirement is the size of your social network." Most retirees are happier if they live close

to friends and family. Some regret moving to a less expensive area because they have to travel extensively to see their family and friends. If you plan to live in the same house at retirement, consider paying off the mortgage by the time you retire.

3. **Health plan** – We're fortunate enough to continue health insurance within the medical group once we retire. But it's important that you invest in yourself by exercising regularly, maintaining a healthy weight, and adopting a sound diet. If you don't have your health, it's difficult to do what's on your bucket list, and your social engagements and other hobbies may be limited.

Step 3: Leave a legacy

1. **Educate your children** – Enroll in a 529 college tuition savings plan. Set one up through Fidelity to help pay for your children's college education.
2. **Assign beneficiaries to your Kaiser Retirement plans** – At Kaiser we also have a life insurance policy that requires a beneficiary's name. At least once a year, review your plan so you know who you plan to leave your Kaiser contribution, your 401k, and your life insurance funds to. If you're having a new child, if you're getting married (or divorced), or if a current beneficiary passes away, it's important to update your beneficiaries.
3. **Consider a living trust** – A trust can transfer your income to family without the headache of probate and the government taking away up to half the estate in

taxes. You will need to contact an estate or tax attorney to help set this up, but it's well worth the expense because you can save your family headaches and money.

I believe that most of us can achieve a financially healthy and personally rewarding retirement. Beyond that, we can all leave a legacy too.

16. Banks and Savings

"If you would be wealthy, think of saving as well as getting."
"An investment in knowledge pays the best interest."

— Benjamin Franklin

When Congress asked Jamie Diamond, CEO of JP Morgan Chase Bank, about his firm's investment strategy if housing prices went down, he said that his bank didn't have one because they didn't think that housing prices would go down. His borrowed money came from individual depositors, like you and me. The money we gave JP Morgan Chase was, by law, insured by the same government asking him the question.

The repeal of the Glass-Steagall Act in 1999 allowed banks to perform both commercial banking and investment banking under one roof. This allowed banks like Citibank, Bank of America, Wells Fargo, and JP Morgan Chase to loan and invest the deposits that we individual investors put into their banks. Banks

Banks and Savings

then made subprime loans with our money, which led to a financial collapse in stock and housing markets.

Charlie Gasparino, a reporter for CNN and the author of the book *Bought and Paid For,* described how subprime mortgages were sold to borrowers unable to repay them. Loans were sold to people, often "qualifying" with no money, no income, and no job (some people called them NINJA loans). Brokers and banks collected commissions when they sold these loans, regardless of whether the loan was ever paid back.

Where do banks get money to loan? Much of it is the savings deposits we put into their banks. Here's the catch: the Federal Deposit Insurance Commission (FDIC) insures our cash deposits up to $250,000, per account. So the money lost by a banks investments (i.e., bad subprime loans or poor stock and bond investments) are insured. How would you like to borrow money and know that if you lost it, Uncle Sam would pay it back to you? That's exactly what happened.

Moral hazard was epidemic as banks risked our money with a government insurance policy. In the end, it was the United States taxpayers (you and I) who "bailed out" big banks for losing our money! The banks got a slap on the hand, then they received checks for billions of dollars, approved by Congress to prevent further collapse of the economy. No, the world is *not* fair.

People who could not repay mortgage loans lost their homes to foreclosure, and the banks got the homes. People were on the street, but bankers got billions in bonuses and bailout money. And banks can still use our deposits to make bad investments because Glass-Steagall is still repealed.

Despite what banks are doing, basic personal finance and saving principals are important in a world of uncertainty. I hope you seriously consider these things when making plans about your personal banking and savings accounts:

1. **Keep an emergency fund (6 – 12 months)** – Save enough living expenses in a non-retirement savings or a money market account. Most banks are relatively safe with our savings because they are FDIC insured up to $250,000 in case your bank goes bankrupt.
2. **Pay off any high-interest credit cards.**
3. **Fund your 401k** – The savings is one of the few government tax breaks to individuals.
4. **Fund an IRA (if you can)** – Even if it's not tax deductible. Beware of the Roth IRA because you need to pay taxes on it to roll over, and in most situations it's better to not pay the tax because most of us use after-tax funds already. We really are double taxed. Ask your accountant.

401k Contribution and Catch-Up Limits*

401k standard contribution limits for 2022 = $20,500

401k catch-up limits for people over fifty for 2022 = $6,500

Current 401k rules allow plan participants who reach the age of fifty before the end of the calendar year to make additional catch-up contributions on a pre-tax basis. As is the case with the "standard" contribution limits, the "catch-up" contribution limits will continue to be indexed for inflation and can increase on a yearly basis in $500 increments.

Banks and Savings

So if you're over the age of fifty in 2022, you can contribute a maximum of $27,000 into a 401k plan.

IRA Contribution and Catch-Up Limits

Traditional IRA limits for 2022 = $6,000

Traditional IRA catch-up limits for people over fifty = $1,000

So if you're over the age of 50 in the year 2022, you can contribute a maximum of $7,000 to a traditional IRA.

The due date for making contributions to an IRA for 2022 is April 17, 2023. In other words, IRA contributions need to be made by the tax due date of the next year.

* Note: I double checked all numbers, but you should always check with your accountant or financial advisor because 401k and IRA limits change, often from year to year.

17. Market Booms and Busts

"An asset bubble is a sort of a natural Ponzi scheme in which people keep making money as long as there are more suckers to draw in. Eventually you run out of suckers and the whole thing crashes."

— Robert Schiller, Case-Schiller Housing Index

I wish I could recognize the next boom so that I can invest just as the market goes up and sell before it collapses. I speculated and bought a house in 2005, near the housing market's peak. I bought it for $200,000 because it was the cheapest place on the water in Clear Lake. The price went up to $230,000, a 15% return. But then the housing market crashed in 2008. Recently, it appraised for $115,000 —ouch! A similar property on the same street sold for $48,000—double ouch! I realize now that I bought in the panic buying phase of a boom-bust cycle.

Since the first reported speculative bubble, the "tulip mania" of 1637, asset booms and busts have become a regular phenomenon in the financial world. In the last decade, two major booms and busts occurred: the stock market e-bubble, which crashed around March of 2000, and the housing bubble, which crashed around October of 2008. After reading economist's John Kenneth Galbraith's book *History of Financial Euphoria* and Charles Mackey's *Extra-ordinary Popular Delusions and the Madness of Crowds*, I have noticed some clear patterns.

The **"boom"** (also known as a **"bubble"**) begins as asset prices increase (e.g., stock prices in the 1990s). This is followed by the **"manic phase,"** when **"panic buying"** often begins (like when I bought the house). Increased values attract new investors, and people often borrow money. This leverage accelerates asset values. Speculators are often inexperienced (like I was when I bought my investment property), and they often buy late and lose big.

Toward the end of the bubble, **"euphoria"** is rampant. According to Schiller's dictum, "The crowd converts the individual of reasonable good sense to stupidity." People may talk of "a new world economy" like they did in 1999, right before the tech market crashed in 2000. Geniuses and the lucky become rich, and the future looks bright just before the bust.

The **"bust"** occurs and the bubble pops when the people who initially rode the wave up start to sell, at first slowly. Then as others see a loss of profits, the selling accelerates. Then pain sets in, and some people sell at any cost to keep what they have. And then **"panic selling"** sets in. People sell, get off margin, stop borrowing, and raise cash. Galbraith wrote, "It always ends not with a whimper, but with a bang." Alan Greenspan once said, "The pain becomes so severe, the only way to relieve it is to sell."

After the bust comes the **"speculative recovery,"** a period when investors regain the confidence—and perhaps the finances—to invest or speculate again. The 1929 stock market crash preceded the Great Depression, and it took the country more than fifteen years to recover. The last part of the cycle—and the beginning of the next boom-bust cycle—is **"speculative dementia,"** a time where people forget the last bust and heal from their economic wounds. This phase is necessary before the next boom-bust cycle starts.

It's interesting how often we humans repeat ourselves. Boom, euphoria, panic buying, panic selling, bust, speculative recovery, dementia—again and again and again. The philosopher George Santayana once wrote, "Those who cannot remember history are doomed to repeat it." I'm hoping that this current speculative recovery in the housing market hurries through the speculative dementia phase and booms again because my lake-side property is under water... financially. Maybe now is actually a good time to buy?

18. Diversification

"The stock market is never obvious. It is designed to fool most of the people, most of the time."

— Jesse Livermore, famous stock trader

Diversification is putting your investments in different stocks, businesses, bonds, real estate, or other investment vehicles. For years, I have spent much of my Sundays looking for stocks and strategies to invest in the market, and I have had a reasonable return in stocks. But spending extraordinary amounts of time learning about those stocks has sometimes felt like a part-time job. Since the recent birth of my son, my time for investing research is now limited (actually, I have no time now). It's hard to justify spending hours and hours on speculation research when I could be parenting.

In 2008, I invested in a company called Hanson, and I spent months following the stock, watching it daily, buying in and out

Diversification

of it, printing out its charts. After about a year—bingo, I nearly doubled my investment. But I could have written several novels in the time it took to study, buy, and sell the stocks. Oh, and I studied about a dozen other stocks, and in spite of that studying and lots of other strategizing besides, my investments lost money that year. I even got a letter from Fidelity that said, "Your recent account activities indicate to us you're a day trader." Let's face it... picking individual stocks is difficult.

Looking for a new strategy that would take less time to pick investments, I arrived at a very sad realization: over the past twenty years, the S&P 500 index had about the same return as the return I was getting from my Sunday-speculation studies. If I'd had spent no more time than what was required to add my 401k funds into the index through a mutual fund or exchange traded fund—which could have been done automatically via payroll deductions—I would have had the same return. Investing in an S&P 500 index would have freed up at least a decade of Sundays. I could have spent more time outside and avoided that dreaded vitamin D deficiency caused by lack of sunshine.

If I had done my homework last year, maybe I would have put all my investment assets into Southwest Airlines (ticker symbol LUV) or Skyworks (SWKS), each of which gained more than a 100% in 2014! But then if I had only invested in the United States Oil (USO) exchange-traded fund that tracks the price of crude oil, my investment would have declined 50% in 2014. And if I had invested all my funds in UWTI—a triple-leveraged, exchange-traded crude oil fund—I would be asking one of you for sleeping pills because UWTI declined from $39 to $2.80 over the course of the year (do the math on this one—it's ugly).

Investment Guide for Doctors

Most investors don't put all their investments in one stock, so the question, then, is this: What portion of our investment portfolios should we put in stocks, bonds, real estate, etc.?

I'll share some of my recent research on ways to save time in retirement investing by focusing on asset allocation. Michael Farr, an investment advisor, who wrote the book *A Million Is Not Enough: How to Retire with the Money You'll Need*, suggests an asset allocation for investors that varies by the investor's age. If a person is just starting out in investing, what he calls a "neo-Boomer," he suggests putting 95% of an investment portfolio in stocks, 4% in bonds, and 1% in cash. He argues that in the long run, stocks will outperform most investments. But if you're a Baby Boomer closer to retirement, he suggests decreasing stock exposure to 60% and investing 30% in bonds and 10% in cash. This recommendation is meant to decrease stock exposure to avoid a massive loss just before retirement. But he also notes that, "Every situation is unique, and these general guidelines are not a one size fits all."

Bob Brinker, an investment advisor who writes a newsletter called *Market Timer*, recommends this asset allocation for aggressive growth investors:

Total stock market fund – 50%
International stock fund – 20%
Small caps fund – 15%
Aggressive growth mutual fund – 15%

John Bogle, the author of *The Little Book of Common Sense Investing* and the inventor of index investing, suggests putting 50% to 95% of our investments in index funds. He says, "If you crave excitement, I would encourage you to do exactly that... but

Diversification

don't invest one penny more than five percent of your investment assets on individual stocks." He calls this a "funny money account."

Jim Cramer, money manager and CNBCs host of *Mad Money*, once said, "After a lifetime of picking stocks, I have to admit that Bogle's arguments in favor of the index fund have me thinking of joining him rather than trying to beat him."

Warren Buffet said, "By periodically investing in an index fund, the know-nothing investor can actually out-perform most investment professionals.... [T]hose index funds are very low cost... investor friendly, and by definition are the best selection for most."

Finances are only a part of life's journey, and most of us would like to see a day when we don't have to work for money, when our time is our own. The truth is that we diversify our time with family, work, and hobbies like working out. Now that I've diversified my time into more family, I've decided to go the simple way and diversify into mostly index funds. I suggest allocating the bulk of your assets in stock investment funds into index funds. Over the long run, they outperform 70% of mutual funds, and that's hard to beat. Allocating investments into indexes allows you to allocate more time to family. Oh, and to work.

Indexed Exchange Traded Funds Ticker Symbols

> **SPY** – "SPYDERS" returns closely follow the S&P 500
> **QQQ** – "Cubes" returns closely follow the Nasdaq, with a high portion of tech stocks
> **DIA** – "DIAMONDS" returns closely follow Dow Jones large-cap funds

19. Getting Good Investment Advice

"The value of market esoterica to the consumer of investment advice is a different story. In my opinion, investment success will not be produced by arcane formula, computer programs or signals flashed by the price behavior of stocks and markets. Rather an investor will succeed by coupling good business judgment with an ability to insulate his thoughts and behavior from the super contagious emotions that swirl about the marketplace."

— Warren Buffett

Most investment advice is a waste of time and money, but investors are still willing to pay for advice, even if it's worthless (I've spent plenty for several investors, and my hope in writing this is that I save you money by helping you learn from my mistakes). No one really knows the direction the stock market will take, but we still pay people to monitor our money through

Getting Good Investment Advice

mutual funds, we attend investment classes, and we subscribe to the magazines and newsletters.

Last fall, I took an investment class from Foothill College to deepen my investment knowledge. A fellow student raised his hand and said, "I have $100,000 to invest. What should I do with it?" The teacher, who owned an investment company, suddenly perked up and told the student to come to his Menlo Park office next week to discuss it. The teachers presented a lot of great ideas in the class, but he was really a salesmen disguised as a teacher, hoping to convert students into clients at his investment firm. And the class cost us $139.

For the past few years, I've watched *Fast Money*, where a panel of professional investors offers opinions. None of them predicted the downturn in the market in 2008. I've also watched Jim Cramer of *Mad Money* for years, and I spent $150 on his three books, which I read, highlighted, and annotated. Then I gave them to Goodwill. I don't watch either of these "free" investment advice shows anymore. Cramer didn't help during the subprime market melt-down either. Bob Brinker missed the 2008 downturn as well, but he's still better than anyone else in the media, in my opinion. He sells a newsletter called *Market Timing*, which I also subscribe to.

I used Gorilla Trades for two years at $500 a year, and I didn't make a dime with their recommended stock picks (of course, I should have followed my own rule: never buy on tips or recommendations.) Gorilla obviously makes money by selling stock picks. One stock the Gorilla suggested dropped 80% the day after he recommended it. Who can afford advice like that?

I subscribed to VectorVest for $650 a year. The yearly subscription runs out in a few months, and I've hardly used their website. I still haven't listened to the five instructional CDs to figure out how to use the system, which is complicated and requires a lot of time to learn. I don't plan to renew it because I have a day job.

Investor's Business Daily is a newspaper that has a proprietary market timing model. It provides daily headlines of business news and a daily interpretation of the stock market. Every Saturday, they publish stocks that might be appropriate for purchase. I still get it, and I plan to renew this summer. It's about $350 a year, and it's available for daily delivery and online. I did a six-month study of the paper's recommended stock picks, and only 17% went up significantly over that period. So I advise caution when purchasing their recommended stocks.

I've subscribed to *Money Magazine* and *Fortune* for several years. *Money Magazine* often gives sound personal financial advice, like starting a Roth IRA, making stock picks, and saving for kids' college. *Fortune Magazine* is better for getting corporate news stories. But I don't recommend either magazine for stock picks.

I've recently read two investment books by medical doctors: *Trading for a Living* ($50, plus $35 for the study guide), written by Hans Elder, M.D., a part-time psychiatrist and stock trader. When I used his strategies, Fidelity sent me a letter warning me that I was a "day trader." I didn't make a dime. Dr. Elder sent me flyers on his trading seminars and information on his proprietary investment software. Then I realized that he was a salesman.

Then I read *Inside the Investors Brain: The Power of Mind over Money*, written by psychiatrists Richard Peterson, M.D. In the book, he mentions a study where most day traders lost 100% of

Getting Good Investment Advice

their money after a year or two. The education was worth the cost of the $50 book, and I stopped trading options. His patients are psychologically troubled investors. He's keeping his day job too.

For me, the real investment lesson was that people giving advice are usually salesman. They know we're desperate for good, honest information, and we're willing to pay for it. Even investment banks make money from the fees they collect when we buy or sell stocks, bonds, or mutual funds, whether or not we make any money. It's a negative-sum game, not a zero-sum game because the broker collects a fee whether we win or lose.

I thought that if I learned enough about the market and kept an eye on it, I would do well. I did bail out before the market crashed in 2009, and I only lost 9% of my investment portfolio, but I had a hard time getting back in. I should have thrown everything in after a good 20% upturn—confirming the bull market—and forgotten about it. Now the market is up 75% from its bottom. Not a single advisor recommended buying stocks or getting back into the market near its low… because they didn't know where the bottom of the market was, and they couldn't predict the new uptrend with any accuracy.

The bottom line is that you're likely better off thinking for yourself. Learning rules and generalizations, studying trends, and acting appropriately to profit. Maybe invest like a contrarian. The old adage says, "Buy low and sell high," but that isn't easy or certain. It *is* the best way to make money in stocks, though.

20. Real Estate Riches: Why Not Become a Slum Lord?

"The only real way to get an education in the market is to invest cash, track your trade and study your mistakes."

— Jesse Livermore, legendary stock trader

A colleague recently asked my advice about buying rental real estate. I'll share my experiences here and offer a little advice.

A good friend's dad worked at IBM and became rich buying real state here in San Jose. His dad bought thirteen houses, then fixed, managed, and rented them. His dad told me, "I'm a damn millionaire." Inspired by my friend's day and by the book *Rich Dad Poor Dad*, I took out a loan and bought a house in Clear Lake Oaks for $200K. The value of the house shot up to $230K, a 15% return in one year. But then during the Great Recession of 2008/2009, the value of the house dropped 65% (yes, that's a $130K loss). But I was undeterred, and I bought another house

Real Estate Riches: Why Not Become a Slum Lord?

because prices were so low. I had two rental properties, and I hired a property manager to rent both houses out.

I had cash flow, but it didn't pay for all my rental expenses, which included the mortgage, homeowner's insurance, property taxes, and (very expensive) flood insurance for two waterfront houses. Then the tenants moved out of one house. The property manager gouged me for $3,000 in repairs. The tenants in the other house stopped paying the water bill, and then stopped paying the rent. I had to hire a lawyer to go to court to put a note on the door to get the non-paying tenants to move out.

I didn't have a property manager or tenants, and I had to pay the bills—all of them. I put the first house up for sale for $75K. I got no offers in six months, so I kept it. Then I hired a new property manager. Currently, I have to pay a small fortune to make the two houses habitable—another out-of-pocket expense.

A few weekends ago, I took my fiancé (a real estate broker and property manager) to visit the rentals in Clear Lake. She noted that there was garbage in front of houses, some of the people in the neighborhood looked like they just gotten out of prison, others looked like they were on their way to drug rehab, and there were motorcycles everywhere. In one of my houses, we found that someone had broken in and stolen the garbage disposable, and an extension cord from the house supplied the next-door neighbor with electricity. On top of all that, the house needed a new roof. My fiancé told me that I was a "slum lord."

My friend's dad and *Rich Dad Poor Dad* now seemed like conversations with drunken pirates looking for buried treasure on an uncharted island. What a mess.

An easier way to invest in real estate without buying and managing properties is to buy real estate–related stocks. Although my two rental houses have lost value, homes in the

Investment Guide for Doctors

Bay Area are up 20% in just the last few years. The real estate market and stock market have both recovered after the Great Recession declines. The S&P 500 index, which represents the largest 500 companies in America, is at an all-time high as of this writing.

Make no mistake, rental real estate is an investment and a business, and sometimes it's very time consuming.

Instead of buying rental real estate—which is difficult to buy and sell quickly and which often requires significant time, repairs, and management commitments—you may want to look at real estate–related stocks. Here are some ideas to consider:

Home Builders

Company Name — Ticker Symbol

KB Home — KBH
Lennar Corp — LEN
The Ryland Group, Inc. — RYL
Toll Brothers, Inc. — TOL

Rental Real Estate Stocks

The Blackstone Group (symbol BLK). According to the 2014 edition of *Money Magazine* they are a "real estate powerhouse" and have "$8 billion to invest in 43,000 homes."

American Homes 4 Rent (symbol AMH) is a real estate

investment trust (REIT), which currently has more than 23,000 single-family properties in twenty-two states.

Home Improvement Stocks

Home Depot (symbol HD)
Lumbar Liquidators (symbol LL)
Lowe's (symbol LOW)

I plan to keep my rental real estate investments, but my experiences as a "slum lord" have convinced me that my next real estate investment will be in real-estate stocks. I told my colleague, who asked for advice, not to buy rental real estate unless you're serious about having a second job and have lots of Excedrin for the headaches that you will encounter. I'm hoping to get two tenants in April to end the rental income drought and help stop the bleeding. In rental real estate, when the bleeding starts and the green dollars turn red, it can be hard to find a financial tourniquet.

21. Savings: The Heart of Investing

"A man with a surplus can control his circumstances, but a man without a surplus is controlled by them, and often has no opportunity to exercise judgment."

— Marshall Field

The first goal of any investment strategy is saving part of what you make each month until you have an emergency fund. The emergency fund should be in cash savings, and it should be enough to cover monthly expenses for six months. Of course it's crucial to know your monthly expense and income.

Your first investment should be creating an emergency fund by saving at least six months of monthly expenses. That requires you to live a bit below your means and put 10% to 20% of your after-tax income into a safe bank account.

Savings: The Heart of Investing

It's important to create an emergency fund before investing a dime in stocks or real estate. The emergency fund should be a key part of everyone's investment strategy.

Emergency funds are important and can help during times of financial stress. It helps when you or your spouse loses a job, when emergency medical bills pop up, when you're hit with unexpected home or vehicle repairs, when you have a tax-time surprise, or when you need travel funds to see a sick family member.

Once you have created a six-month emergency fund, you should start investing in retirement accounts. That's a 401k or an IRA for most of us. The 401k is deducted pre-tax from our paychecks each month, and if you haven't signed up yet, it's a must. An IRA likely isn't tax deductible, but the funds grow tax free, and I suggest starting one because gains aren't taxed until you make withdrawals.

Another reason to consider a savings fund is because stock market returns aren't always positive. According to investment writer Doug Short, since the stock market peak in 2000, the S&P 500 return has been -30%, the Dow -15%, and the Nasdaq -54%. That's right, all the major stock market indexes have negative returns today from the stock markets' peak in 2000. Some call this the lost decade of investing.

In the past decade, we have lived through two stock market crashes of more than 50%: the tech bubble of 2000 and the financial crises of 2009. Given all the volatility, I think it's very important to have a cash savings emergency fund. That money won't be lost in the stock market, and, more importantly, it can help improve your sleep at night, knowing that you have a safety net.

It may be the case that saving money in the bank since the market peak in 2000 would have resulted in a better return than investing in the market because there would be no loss of your investment principle.

Seven Healthy Financial Habits

1. Pay yourself first
2. Save your tax refund and any work bonuses
3. Cut back on your personal expenses
4. Set a savings goal
5. Turn savings into a game
6. Put extra cash or savings into a jar
7. Make savings a habit

22. Spending Power: Personal Finance 101

"Annual income twenty pounds, annual expenditure nineteen six, result happiness. Annual income twenty pounds, annual expenditure twenty pound ought and six, result misery."

— Charles Dickens

Schools usually don't teach personal finance. Parents sometimes teach it, but, unfortunately, conversations about money are often taboo in many families. As Congress debates our country's budget and decides whether to raise the debt ceiling, I thought it appropriate to review some ideas of basic personal finance and the concept of spending power.

I had my first experience with budgeting and personal finance the year I worked as a lab tech after graduating from college, before going to medical school. I earned a whopping $13,000 for the entire year, more money than I had ever seen in my entire life. The first six months were great. I went out and had a lot of pizza and beer with my friends, and I didn't save a penny.

Something's wrong, I thought. So, I picked up *The Only Investment Guide You'll Ever Need*, a book by Andrew Tobias. It was the first investment book I ever read. The most important lesson was that he recommended putting 10% to 20% of each paycheck into your savings account and pretending that it doesn't exist, and he advised living on the rest.

After reading that book—religiously—I started putting 10% to 20% of each paycheck into savings. My lifestyle didn't change at all. The only thing that changed was my savings account. In the second six months, I had saved more than $1,500. Trying to save 10% to 20% of each paycheck was the book's most important lesson. In the book *The Richest Man in Babylon*, George Samuel Clason writes that "part of what you earn is yours to keep." That's how I tried to live.

Today, not much has changed, except things are more complicated—credit cards, house payments, 401k's, rental properties, brokerage accounts, etc. Ensuring that income minus expenses is a positive number each month is still important. Most people who win millions in the lottery lose all their money or go bankrupt because they never had a system to manage it properly in the first place.

> **Ensuring that income minus expenses is a positive number each month is still important.**

CPA Robert Ortlada's book *Financial Sanity* uses the term **"spending power,"** which is monthly income minus expenses. Spending power is the amount of money left over each month for additional debt reduction, vacations, second homes, etc.

after you cover all your regular expenses, including 401k deductions.

Spending power = monthly income - monthly expenses

It's pretty easy to calculate your spending power if your income and expenses are in one checking account. Each month, add up all the income in the account (use after-tax income) and subtract it from all the expenses. The goal is to have a positive number each month. Anyone serious about keeping track can set up a spreadsheet and keep a monthly tally of income and expenses. After you subtract expenses from income, you have your spending power. If the number is negative, you should explore your expenses because you're likely living beyond your means, and that could mean financial trouble. Making it a habit of calculating your spending power once a month isn't very cumbersome, especially if your income and expenses are in one checking account.

One issue that will come up is major yearly expenses like property taxes and home and auto insurances. Look back at last year's major expenses and add them up, then divide by 12. Each month, put that amount into a separate savings account, and take it out to pay the bulk expense when it comes due.

Consistency in calculating spending power is a vital tool in your personal finance toolbox. It will help you manage debt and know whether you can afford a new investment or expense. Calculating it monthly and putting it on a spreadsheet allows you to go back and see how you're doing from month to month. At the end of the year, you can go back and determine your average income and your average expenses for the year, which helps you set a budget for the upcoming year. It may help to set aside time at the beginning of each month to make that calculation.

Whatever your method for tracking your personal finances, I hope you calculate your spending power. Never forget that "a part of what you earn is yours to keep," but you have to know if there's something left after you have paid your expenses.

Andrew Tobias, author of *The Only Investment Guide You'll Ever Need*, wrote that there are several things "screaming to be done." They include:

1. 401k—contribute to the maximum
2. Put as much savings into an IRA as possible, even if it's tax deductible
3. Have some equity in your home
4. Have $1,000 for bulk purchases
5. Increase the deductible in your home and automobile insurance
6. Pay off all 18% credit cards (financially healthy people pay them off monthly)
7. Save at least 10% to 20% of each paycheck (this can include a pre-tax 401k account, kids' college funds, an IRA, savings to a brokerage account, or just savings)

23. Can Decluttering Make You Wealthy?

"I like material things as much as anyone. I studied product design in school. I'm into gadgets, clothing and all kinds of things. But my experiences show that after a certain point, material objects have a tendency to crowd out the emotional needs they are meant to support."

— Graham Hill, *NY Times* article

"Any half-awake materialist well knows—that which you hold holds you."

—Tom Robbins

Many people believe that downsizing to a smaller home at retirement is a wise financial move. The idea, as I understand it, is that we sell our home and use the equity to purchase a less expensive home outright. Then in retirement, we have no monthly mortgage. In other words, the only housing expenses other than maintenance are property taxes and home insurance, a mere pittance compared to the cost of a monthly thirty-year mortgage payment.

Paying cash for a less expensive home helps you avoid that monthly mortgage payment, but most people will have to move out of the Silicon Valley to find a less expensive neighborhood. But in the book *Retire Happy*, the authors suggest that a social life is the most rewarding part of retirement. I have taken a (very unofficial) poll, mostly among my patients. Many move and downsize, but they keep returning to the Bay Area to see their family and friends.

One couple moved from San Jose to parts unknown. The best description of the location was "many miles south of Lake Tahoe." Their place got snowed in during the winter, but she and her husband were introverts, so they didn't care about being around people. They loved it. Another couple moved to Sacramento and hated it because she couldn't see her children and grandkids as often. Yet another patient came in anxious and depressed because his daughter was moving out of the Bay Area, taking his grandkids to Idaho. He said, "Maybe I'll move out to be with her when I retire in three years."

Before you decide, ask yourself this: Do I want to retire in a place near my family and friends so I can maintain my social interactions, or do I want to move to a less-expensive location where it would be more difficult to stay in contact with family and friends? Even if you know the answer, I suggest that you declutter your current living situation. The rewards are great now, and they can pay dividends when you retire.

Years ago, I read Suzie Orman's book *The Courage to Be Rich*. A chapter called "The Courage to Make Room for More Money" really struck me. She suggested that we declutter our minds and recognize that "emotional obstacles—shame, fear, anger—stand between us and more.... Clear away the internal clutter." That clutter can hold us back from our desires. As she explains, "The last obstacle that must be cleared away is the material clutter: the sheer volume of items in your life that you no longer value and no longer need."

Two years ago, I took this message to heart after I looked for a pair of scissors, some string, and a book, all of which I had in my house but none of which I could find. Instead of spending an hour looking for the tape, scissors, and book, I purchased these "inexpensive" items again, adding to my clutter. Eventually, I realized that after nearly twenty years of living in the same house, it was time for me to declutter so I could find things.

Then I did what Suzie Orman recommended: I went through the house and found items I could throw away or give to Goodwill. I had a few thousand books, hundreds of CDs, nearly twenty pairs of shoes (when I was a child, my family survived on welfare, and I had only one pair of shoes at a time. I wore them until they had holes in them), and a collection of baseball cards (I'm embarrassed to tell you the number I had collected over the years, all gathered in boxes in the garage). But what to do with all these items? I realized it was probably the childhood poverty that was making me hang on to those collections. Suzie Orman's book gave me a jumpstart, but I still couldn't bring myself to declutter significantly to reap the rewards.

Then I read the book *The Life-Changing Magic of Tidying Up* by Marie Condo. She suggests undertaking an intensive discarding program of getting rid of things that you don't use. Instead of a moderate decluttering, she suggested taking a more radical approach, explaining, "Dramatic reorganization of the home causes correspondingly dramatic changes in lifestyle and perspective. It is life transforming." It was difficult at first, but a strange transition occurred in me as I "cleansed" the house, paring down my collection of books to about 100, my CDs to about fifty, my shoes to six pairs, and my baseball cards from ten boxes to two.

I made at least ten trips to Goodwill and donated books to the library, recirculating things no longer in use in my house. Months later, I could easily find a pair of scissors, some string, and a book. I could even find my financial records and could keep tabs of my monthly finances with more clarity. I didn't stop there. I took out furniture, bookcases, CD cases, extra chairs, and an old chest of drawers in the guest room. I felt lighter, my mind less cluttered. I treasured and appreciated the things I owned and the house that I lived in more than I had in years.

Even though I loved the house, I thought about downsizing to a smaller place. Not that I wanted to retire or move out of the area. I love my job and the people I work with. I talked with a Realtor and found a smaller home with a nice view, close to the office. When the new home closed, the move was much easier because I had already decluttered. I took only items that I loved from the old house to the new one, but the new house was smaller, so I needed to downsize even more.

After four months of living in the new smaller home, I hadn't even put a nail to hang a picture on the wall, and I felt that I needed to clear out more things. I made another twelve trips to Goodwill and pared down my collections even more. I searched online and discovered a minimalist movement. I read Jay Francine's book *The Joy of Less: A Minimalist Living Guide*. She promised all of the following benefits of decluttering:

- Less stuff = less stress
- Less stuff = less pressure to consume
- Less stuff = less to clean
- Less stuff = more freedom
- Less stuff = more money
- Less stuff = more time
- Less stuff = more joy

Wow! That's a lot of promises for decluttering our homes and having less stuff.

In the end, decluttering helped me learn to appreciate my home more, it seemed to open up space physically and mentally for new and good things in my life, and I believe it allowed me to move to a nicer home. Although smaller, the home I moved to actually cost more than the previous one. But it's a place I would be happy to retire in, where I can stay close to friends and family in the Bay Area. In my mind, it just begs the question: When I retire, why would I want to move and have to clean all my stuff out again? The truth is that I could clean out my stuff, declutter, and get rid of the things I don't cherish. That would make space for treasures in my life.

Make space for the new now, before retirement. If you plan to move and "downsize," you have already had practice and experience. Understanding that decluttering can make us wealthy isn't rocket science. Making space, clearing clutter, and keeping only what I treasure has given me more than the promised wealth. The reward has been priceless. It brought peace of mind—and now I can even find a pair of scissors.

About the Author

Steve Petty enjoys music, sports, teaching, and travel. He is a primary care physician in San Jose, California; graduated from the Medical School at the University of California, Irvine; and trained at the San Jose Family Practice Residency, which is affiliated with Stanford University. He is board certified in both family medicine and sports medicine. Steve has spent over fifteen years as an adjunct clinical assistant professor at Stanford Medical School's Department of Family Medicine. He also writes a quarterly investment column.

Other Books by the Author

Affirmations: Guides to Feel Good About Yourself
Famous Doctors: A Brief Biography of Medicine
Petty Therapy Song Book
Poetry: A Young Life in Poems
The Allergy Epidemic: Understanding and Treating Environmental Allergies
Student Doctor: Surviving and Thriving in Medical School

Music CDs by the Author

It's a Good Life
I Want to Sing
Live at 9 Lives Club
Love Songs
Silicon Valley Blues
Take This Monkey off My Back

All Steve's books and CDs are available on Amazon.com. His author page is *Amazon.com/author/stevepettymd*

www.ingramcontent.com/pod-product-compliance
Lightning Source LLC
Chambersburg PA
CBHW071422210526
45465CB00001B/491